INTERMITTENT
FASTING COOKBOOK

QUICK AND EASY RECIPES TO LOSE WEIGHT, UNLOCK YOUR
METABOLISM, AND REJUVENATE YOUR BODY

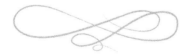

Mary Light

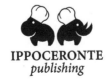

IPPOCERONTE
publishing

Contents

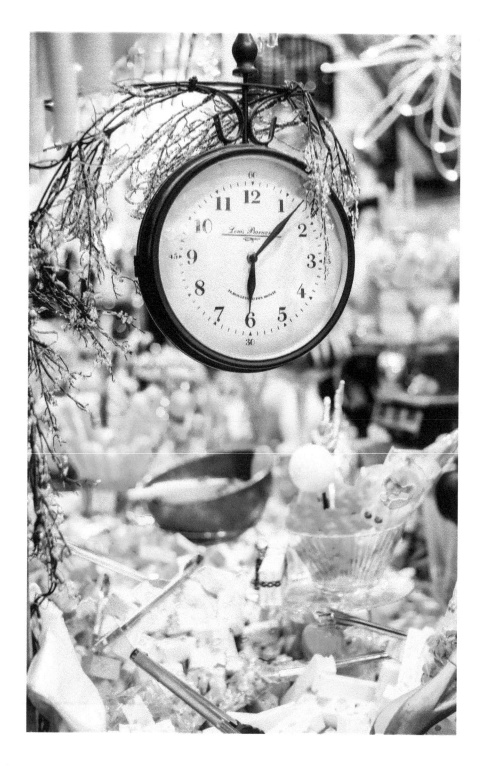

Introduction

Intermittent fasting has several advantages that make it ideal for women as they age. Not only do women struggle to lose weight as their metabolism slows as they age, but they are also more susceptible to a variety of age- and weight-related ailments. We'll go over some of the best reasons to choose this lifestyle in detail. This will allow you to determine if it is a good fit for you.

The first advantage of intermittent fasting is that it helps you feel full while eating less food. Studies show that intermittent fasting helps to shed pounds and reduce belly fat in roughly equal measure. By avoiding the constant need to eat, this diet minimizes the chances of overeating or feeling dissatisfied with your food. Forcing yourself to eat smaller portions, especially at breakfast when your appetite tends to be the strongest, is a surefire way to lose weight.

Weight Loss

While many people attempt diet after diet in the hopes of losing weight, they are more likely to succeed with intermittent fasting. After all, while the human body is normally forced to burn off the food we have eaten on a regular basis, when you are fasted, you can work on burning off your body fat instead.

Metabolic Reset

Many women, as they age, experience reduced metabolism. The best way to correct this is by resetting your metabolism, which is exactly what intermittent fasting does. For those unfamiliar with the concept of metabolism, it is the way that your body uses food for energy. Intermittent fasting allows you to reduce both of these actions, so you have less stored body fat and more usable energy from food.

Intermittent fasting has several advantages that make it ideal for women as they age. Not only do women struggle to lose weight as their metabolism slows as they age, but they are also more susceptible to a variety of age- and weight-related ailments. We'll go over some of the best reasons to choose this lifestyle in detail. This will allow you to determine if it is a good fit for you.

The first advantage of intermittent fasting is that it helps you feel full while eating less food. Studies show that intermittent fasting helps to shed pounds and reduce belly fat in roughly equal measure. By avoiding the constant need to eat, this diet minimizes the chances of overeating or feeling dissatisfied with your food.

Forcing yourself to eat smaller portions, especially at breakfast when your appetite tends to be the strongest, is a surefire way to lose weight.

INCREASE HUMAN GROWTH HORMONE

HGH, or Human Growth Hormone, is a hormone that many people lose as they get older. Although many other hormones decline as you get older, this is one that you can actively improve by making small lifestyle changes. During your fast, you will take extra doses of this hormone to help repair your worn and damaged tissues.

CONVERT YOUR BODY FAT

When you fast, your body is able to burn body fat much more effectively than when you eat. This is due to the fact that most of our body's cells are unable to use glucose as a primary energy source because they are often working while you sleep and lack the energy to exercise. Intermittent fasting allows your cells to use fat for fuel, which results in weight loss.

IMPROVE MUSCLE HEALTH

When you are fasting, your body does not have the resources to work out as many times per week as it would if you were eating. While your muscles do not rely on glucose for energy, they do rely on protein for a greater portion of their requirements. Fasting allows your body to more effectively use stored protein to produce the energy required by your muscles, making them stronger and healthier.

BOOSTED ENERGY

You may find that when you fast, your energy levels are much higher than when you eat. The reason for this is that fasting burns glucose out of your system, preventing it from being used as a source of energy. When you're hungry, you'll be compelled to look for food rather than take on the task of burning off the sugar in your body. This leads to more coherent and optimal energy levels throughout the day, as well as a healthier lifestyle overall.

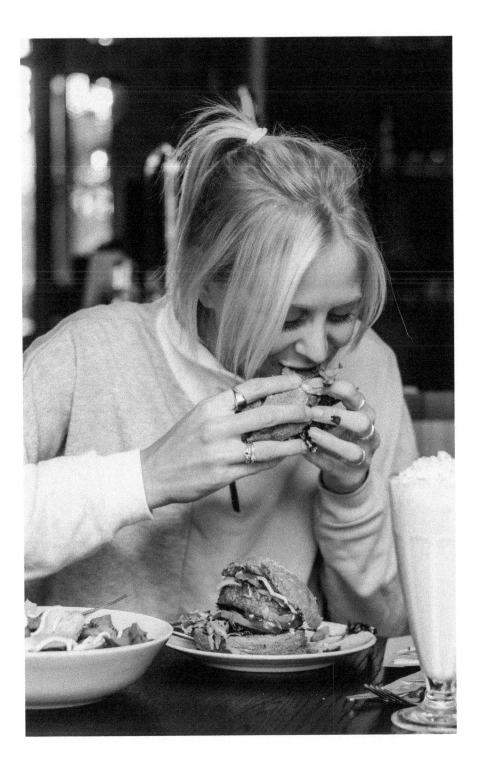

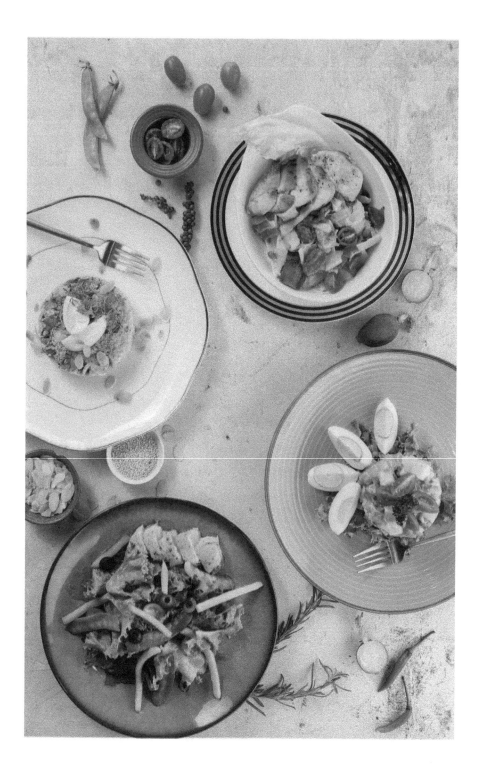

RECIPES

1. GRILLED PROSCIUTTO WRAPPED ASPARAGUS

Cal.: 50 | Fat: 2.5g | Protein: 4g

Preparation Time: 5 minutes
Cooking Time: 10 minutes
Servings: 4

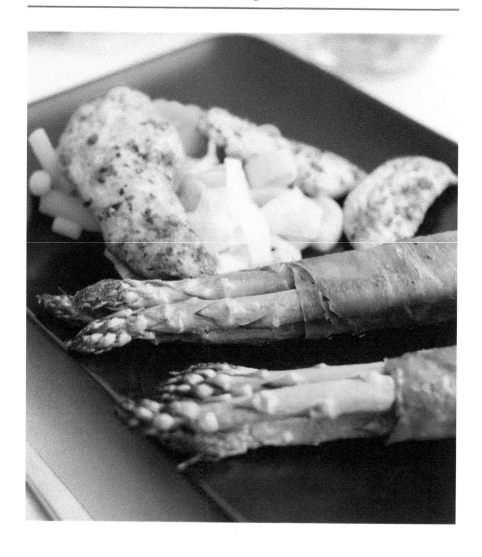

Ingredients

16 asparagus spears, rimmed at the ends
4 slices Prosciutto
Olive oil for greasing
Kosher salt for tasting
Black pepper for tasting

Directions

1. Cut each piece of prosciutto into 4 pieces and wrap each piece around the center of each spear.

2. Spritz with olive oil, season the asparagus tips with a pinch of salt and season the rest with black pepper.

3. Light the grill over light heat, when hot clean and oil the grates.

4. Grill the asparagus 5 to 6 minutes, covered on low turning every few minutes

2. CHEESY TACO SKILLET

Cal.: 287 | Fat: 8g | Protein: 28g

Preparation Time: 10 minutes
Cooking Time: 20 minutes
Servings: 4

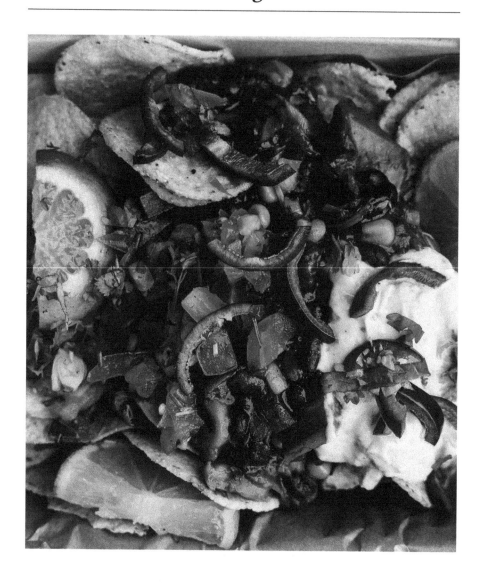

Ingredients

1 pound of lean grass-fed ground beef
1 large yellow or white onions, finely chopped
2 medium-sized bell peppers, finely chopped
1 (12-ounce) can of diced tomatoes with green chilis
2 large zucchinis, finely chopped
2 tablespoons of taco seasoning
3 cups of fresh baby kale or fresh spinach
1 ½ cups of shredded cheddar cheese OR shredded jack cheese

Directions

1. In a large nonstick skillet, add the ground beef and cook until lightly brown. Drain the excess grease.

2. Add the chopped onions, chopped bell peppers, diced tomatoes with green chilis, zucchini, and taco seasoning. Cook for 5 minutes, stirring occasionally.

3. Add the fresh baby kale or spinach. Cook until wilted.

4. Cover with 1 ½ cups of shredded cheddar cheese and cover with a lid.

5. Once the cheese has melted, serve and enjoy!

3. BACON EGG & SAUSAGE CUPS

Cal.: 100 | Fat: 8g | Protein: 5g

Preparation Time: 10 minutes
Cooking Time: 20 minutes
Servings: 8

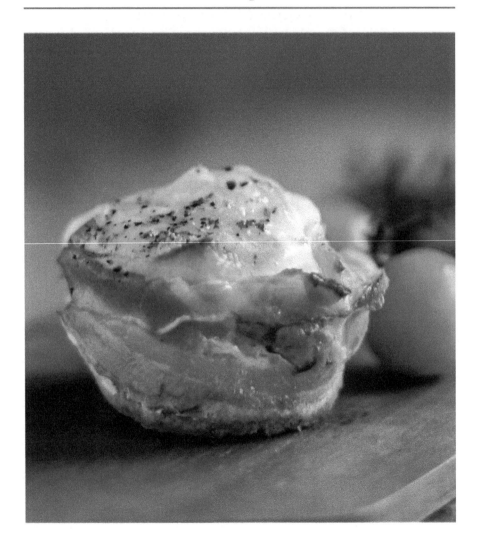

Ingredients

3 oz. breakfast sausages
2 slices bacon, chopped
4 large eggs
2 large green onions, chopped
1 oz. cheddar cheese, shredded
1 tbsp. coconut oil

Directions

1. Preheat the oven to 350°F. Grease your muffin pan and set aside.

2. In a mixing bowl, beat the eggs together with the cheese. Set aside.

3. Brown the bacon in a non-stick skillet over medium heat. Add the crumbled sausage and cook until no longer pink.

4. Add the onion and cook until wilted. Remove the skillet from the heat and let it cool for a minute or two. Add the meat mixture to the egg mixture and beat well using a spoon.

5. Scoop mixture into the greased muffin pan and bake for 15-20 minutes or until the tops begin to brown. Remove from pan and serve.

4. SPINACH SAMOSA

Cal.: 254 | Fat: 12.2g | Protein: 10.2g

Preparation Time: 15 minutes
Cooking Time: 15 minutes
Servings: 2
Requirements: Air fryer

Ingredients

1 ½ cups of almond flour
½ teaspoon baking soda
1 teaspoon garam masala
1 teaspoon coriander, chopped
¼ cup green peas
½ teaspoon sesame seeds
¼ cup potatoes, boiled, small chunks
2 tablespoons olive oil
¾ cup boiled and blended spinach puree
Salt and chili powder to taste

Directions

1. In a bowl, mix baking soda, salt, and flour to make the dough. Add 1 tablespoon of oil. Add the spinach puree and mix until the dough is smooth.

2. Place in the fridge for 20 minutes.

3. In the pan add one tablespoon of oil, then add potatoes, peas and cook for 5 minutes. Add the sesame seeds, garam masala, coriander, and stir.

4. Knead the dough and make the small ball using a rolling pin. Form balls, make into cone shapes, which are then filled with stuffing that is not yet fully cooked. Make sure flour sheets are well sealed.

5. Preheat the air fryer to 390° F. Place samosa in the air fryer basket and cook for 10 minutes.

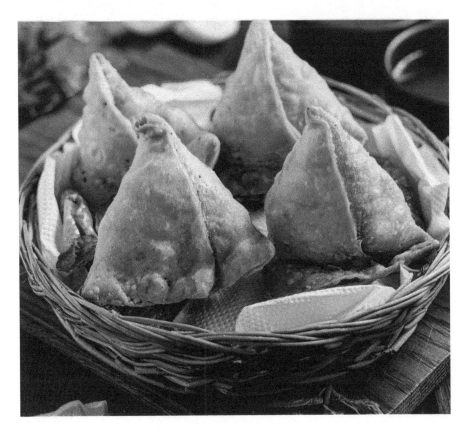

5. SESAME-SEARED SALMON

Cal.: 198 | Fat: 12g | Protein: 5g

Preparation Time: 5 minutes
Cooking Time: 10 minutes
Servings: 4

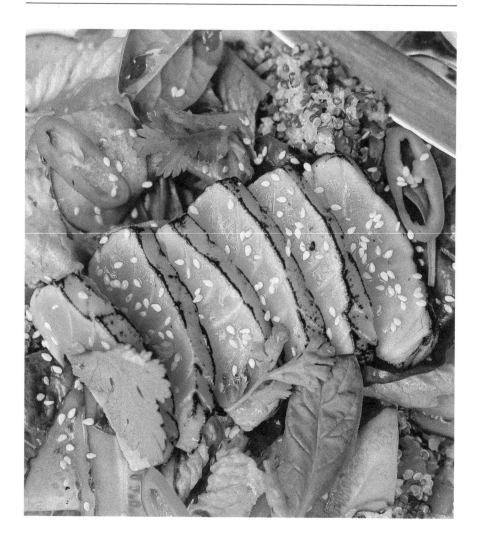

Ingredients

4 wild salmon fillets (about 1lb.)
1½ tbsps. Sesame seeds
2 tbsps. Toasted sesame oil
1½ tbsps. Avocado oil
1 tsp. sea salt

Directions

1. Using a paper towel or a clean kitchen towel, pat the fillets to dry. Brush each with a tablespoon of sesame oil and season with a half teaspoon of salt.

2. Place a large skillet over medium-high heat and drizzle with avocado oil. Once the oil is hot, add the salmon fillets with the flesh side down. Cook for about 3 minutes and flip. Cook the skin side for an additional 3-4 minutes, without overcooking it.

3. Remove the pan from the heat and brush with the remaining sesame oil. Season with the remaining salt and sprinkle with sesame seeds. Best served with green salad.

6. PORK CARNITAS

Cal.: 294 | Fat: 12g | Protein: 45g

Preparation Time: 10 minutes
Cooking Time: 50 minutes
Servings: 4

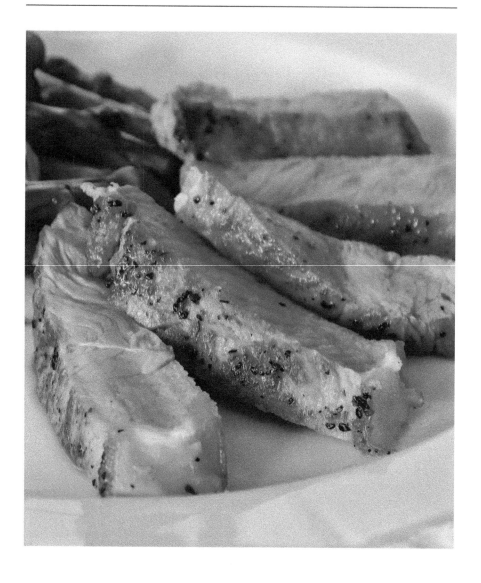

Ingredients

Pepper
0.25 tsp. Salt
0.5 tbsp. Dark molasses
0.5 tbsp. Orange juice
1 tbsp. Brown sugar
1 Minced garlic clove
0.5 lb. Pork tenderloin

Directions

1. Rinse off the pork tenderloin and blot it down with some paper towels. Slice thinly and then set it aside.

2. Place a skillet on a flame or burner set to high, and then heat it up for about a minute. Once the skillet is hot, add the pork tenderloin. Cook these for about 4 minutes until the pork is tender and cooked throughout.

3. Drain out the oil before stirring in the pepper, salt, molasses, orange juice, and brown sugar.

4. Stir this around and simmer until your sauce is thick. Turn off the heat and let it stand for a few minutes to thicken before serving.

7. MINI THAI LAMB SALAD BITES

Cal.: 58 | Fat: 2g | Protein: 5g

**Preparation Time: 10 minutes
Cooking Time: 8 minutes
Servings: 15**

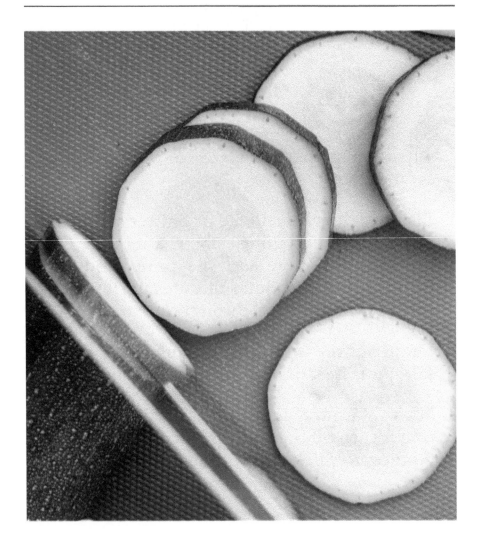

Ingredients

1 large cucumber, cut into 0.39-inch-thick
diagonal rounds
0.55 lb. (250g) Lamb Backstrap
3/4 cup Cherry Tomatoes, quartered
1/3 cup fresh mint, loosely packed
1/3 cup fresh coriander, loosely packed
1/4 small red onion, finely diced
1 tsp. fish sauce
Juice of 1 lime
Coconut oil

Directions

1. Place the pan over medium heat and heat oil.
   Cook the lamb for 4 minutes on each side.
   Remove from heat and let it rest.

2. In a mixing bowl, toss the onions, tomatoes,
   mint, coriander, fish sauce, and lime juice.

3. Cut the lamb into thin strips and add to the
   salad bowl. Toss to combine.

4. Spoon ample amounts of mixture on each
   cucumber cut. Chill and serve.

8. STUFFED PORTOBELLO MUSHROOMS

Cal.: 320 | Fat: 8g | Protein: 34g

Preparation Time: 10 minutes
Cooking Time: 20 minutes
Servings: 4

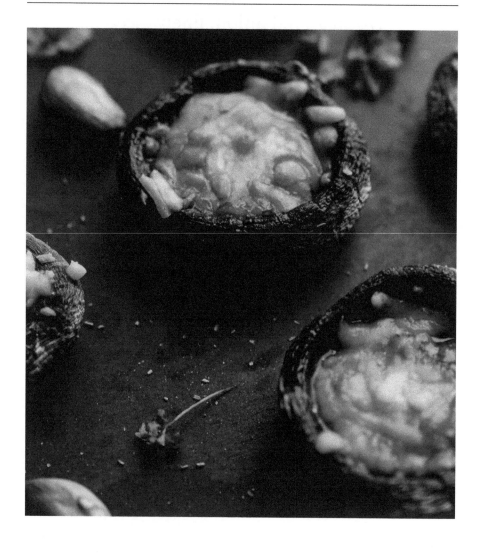

Ingredients

8 portobello mushrooms, the large ones are best
6oz kale, the fresher the better
8 slices of cheese, go for the one you like more
2 tbsp olive oil, extra virgin is best here also

Directions

1. Preheat your oven to 250C

2. Take a baking sheet and cover with parchment paper

3. Place the mushrooms onto the tray, with the 'cup' facing upwards

4. Drizzle a little of the olive oil over the top of the mushrooms and place in the oven for around 10 minutes

5. Once cooked, add a slice of cheese to each mushroom and a little of the cake

6. Place back in the oven for another 3 minutes; the mushrooms are cooked when the cheese is melted and bubbling

7. Allow cooling a little before serving

9. GROUND BEEF AND CAULIFLOWER HASH

Cal.: 311 | Fat: 7g | Protein: 33g

Preparation Time: 10 minutes
Cooking Time: 25 minutes
Servings: 6

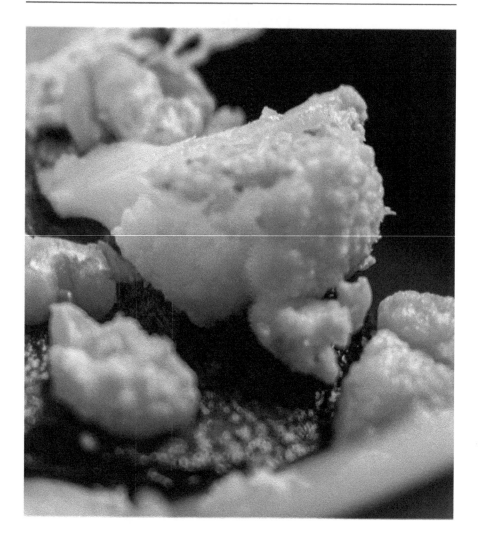

Ingredients

1 (16-ounce) bag of frozen cauliflower florets,
defrosted and drained
1 pound of lean grass-fed ground beef
2 cups of shredded cheddar cheese
1 teaspoon of garlic powder
½ teaspoon of fine sea salt
½ teaspoon of freshly cracked black pepper

Directions

1. In a large skillet over medium-high heat, add the ground beef and cook until brown. Drain the excess grease.

2. Add the cauliflower florets, garlic powder, fine sea salt and freshly cracked black pepper. Cook until the cauliflower is tender, stirring occasionally.

3. Add the shredded cheddar cheese to the cauliflower and ground beef mixture.

4. Remove from the heat and cover with a lid. Allow the steam to melt the cheese.

5. Serve and enjoy!

10. SMOKED SALMON & AVOCADO STACKS

Cal.: 106 | Fat: 12g | Protein: 5g

Preparation Time: 15 minutes
Cooking Time: 0 minutes
Servings: 6

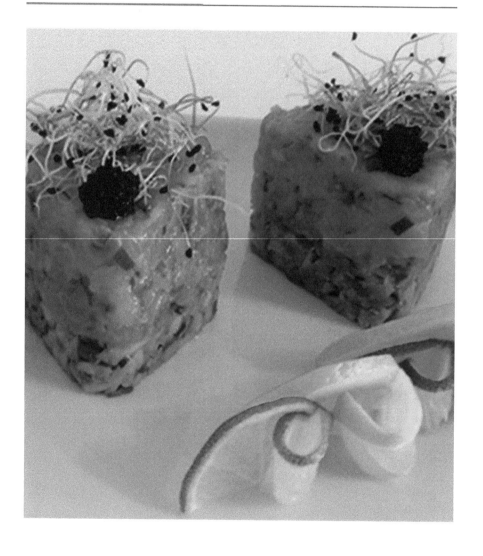

Ingredients

½ lb. smoked salmon, finely diced
1 ripe avocado, seed removed and diced
1 tbsp. chives, chopped
Fresh or dried dill leaves
3 tsps. fresh lemon juice
Black pepper, cracked

Directions

1. Combine salmon, chives, and a teaspoon of lemon juice in a small mixing bowl.

2. In another mixing bowl, toss the avocado, remaining lemon juice, and pepper.

3. Using a presentation ring, arrange the stacks on the serving plates. Arrange the avocado at the bottom and top it with the salmon mixture and gently press. Remove the mold and garnish the stack with dill leaves. Serve chilled.

11. QUICK RATATOUILLE

Cal.: 270 | Fat: 8g | Protein: 6g

Preparation Time: 10 minutes
Cooking Time: 12 minutes
Servings: 4

Ingredients

2 onions, sliced
4 cloves of garlic, chopped very finely
0.5 cup olive oil
1 green pepper, cut into small pieces
1 red pepper, cut into small pieces
1 aubergine (eggplant), cut into cubes
4 zucchinis, cubed
8 tomatoes, seeded and chopped
1 tbsp basil, shredded. Fresh is best but if you
have to go with dried, just use 1 tsp)
1.5 tsp salt
A little black pepper

Directions

1. You will need a large and deep-frying pan or saucepan,

2. Add the oil and allow to reach a medium to high heat

3. Add the onions and the garlic and cook for a few minutes, until the onions are clear

4. Add the peppers, zucchini, and the aborigine (eggplant) and combine

5. Turn the heat down and play an over the pan, allowing it to simmer for around 10 minutes

6. Add the salt and pepper, as well as the tomatoes and stir well, covering the pan once more and allowing it to continue cooking for another 10 minutes

7. Take the lid off the pan and stir the mixture, allowing it to reduce

8. Add a little salt and pepper and serve whilst still warm. The mixture is done when it is blended well, but isn't particularly 'wet'

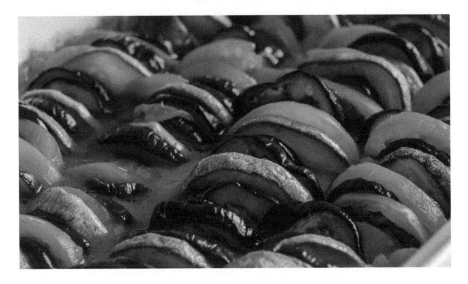

12. PASTA BOLOGNESE SOUP

Cal.: 182 | Fat: 4g | Protein: 3g

Preparation Time: 10 minutes
Cooking Time: 35 minutes
Servings: 5

Ingredients

2 tsp olive oil
3 onions, chopped finely
2 carrots, peeled and chopped finely
2 celery stick, chopped finely
3 cloves of garlic, chopped finely
250g of lean steak/beef mince
500g pasta
1 tbsp vegetable stock
1 tsp paprika, smoked works well
4 pieces of thyme, fresh
100mg penne, whole meal
45g parmesan cheese, grated finely

Directions

1. Take a large pan and add the oil, heat over a medium heat

2. Add the onions and cook until translucent

3. Add the carrots, garlic, and the celery, cooking for 5 minutes

4. Add the mince to the pan and break it up well

5. Once the mince has browned, add the stock and the passata, adding 1 liter of hot water

6. Stir well and then add the thyme and paprika, combining once more

7. Add the lid to the pan and allow to simmer for 15 minutes

8. Add the penne and stir through, cooking for another 165 minutes

9. Add the cheese and stir

10.　Serve in bowls whilst still warm

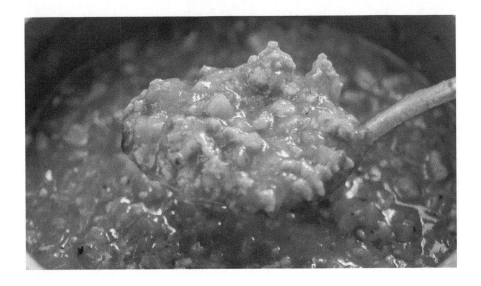

13. TURKEY WALNUT SALAD

Cal.: 390 | Fat: 4g | Protein: 56g

Preparation Time: 10 minutes
Cooking Time: 50 minutes
Servings: 4

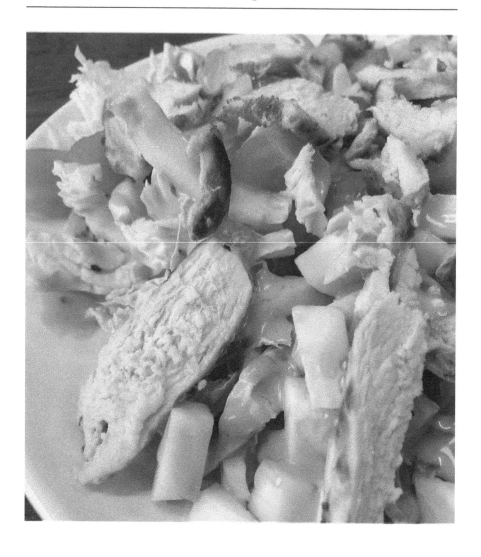

Ingredients

0.25 cup Chopped walnuts
1 Chopped celery
0.5 pc. Chopped yellow onion
8 oz. Minced turkey
Pepper
Salt
2 tsp. Parsley
1 tsp. Lemon juice
1 tbsp. Dijon mustard
2 tbsps. Greek yogurt
2 tbsps. Mayo
3 tbsps. Dried cranberries

Directions

1. Take out a bowl and combine the cranberries, walnuts, celery, onion, and turkey.

2. In another bowl, combine the pepper, salt, parsley, lemon juice, mustard, Greek yogurt, and mayo.

3. Combine both bowls together and toss well to mix evenly before serving.

14. EASY ITALIAN ZUCCHINI FRITTERS

Cal.: 127 | Fat: 6g | Protein: 10g

Preparation Time: 15 minutes
Cooking Time: 20 minutes
Servings: 6

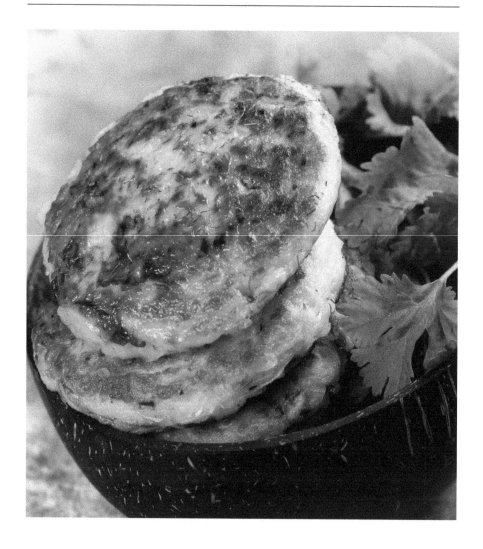

Ingredients

4 cloves minced garlic
1 teaspoon sea salt
2 large eggs
2 teaspoons Italian seasoning
8 cups grated zucchini
1 cup parmesan cheese, grated
Olive oil to fry with

Directions

1. Place the zucchini and salt into a large colander and mix together. Drain over the sink for 10 minutes.

2. Wrap the zucchini in a kitchen towel. Squeeze and twist over the sink to drain as much water as possible.

3. Place the zucchini into a large bowl. Add remaining ingredients and stir them together.

4. Heat a generous amount of olive oil in a large skillet over medium-high heat for about 2 minutes. Spoon rounded tablespoonfuls (28 grams) of the batter onto the skillet and flatten to about 1/4 to 1/3 inch thick. Fry for about 2 minutes on each side until golden brown.

5. Serve with sour cream and parsley.

15. CRISPY BLACK-EYED PEAS

Cal.: 262 | Fat: 9.4g | Protein: 9.2g

Preparation Time: 10 minutes
Cooking Time: 15 minutes
Servings: 6

Ingredients

15 ounces black-eyed peas
1/8 teaspoon chipotle chili powder
¼ teaspoon salt
½ teaspoon chili powder
1/8 teaspoon black pepper

Directions

1. Rinse the beans well with running water then set aside.

2. In a large bowl, mix the spices until well combined. Add the peas to spices and mix.

3. Place the peas in the wire basket and cook for 10 minutes at 360° F.

4. Serve and enjoy!

16. LEMONY GREEN BEANS

Cal.: 263 | Fat: 9.2g | Protein: 8.7g

Preparation Time: 12 minutes
Cooking Time: 15 minutes
Servings: 4
Requirements: Air fryer

Ingredients

1 lb. green beans washed and destemmed
Sea salt and black pepper to taste
1 lemon
¼ teaspoon extra virgin olive oil

Directions

1. Preheat your air fryer to 400° F. Place the green beans in the air fryer basket.

2. Squeeze lemon over beans and season with salt and pepper.

3. Cover ingredients with oil and toss well.

4. Cook green beans for 12 minutes and serve!

17. ROASTED ORANGE CAULIFLOWER

Cal.: 344 | Fat: 21g | Protein: 19g

Preparation Time: 20 minutes
Cooking Time: 15 minutes
Servings: 2
Requirements: Air fryer

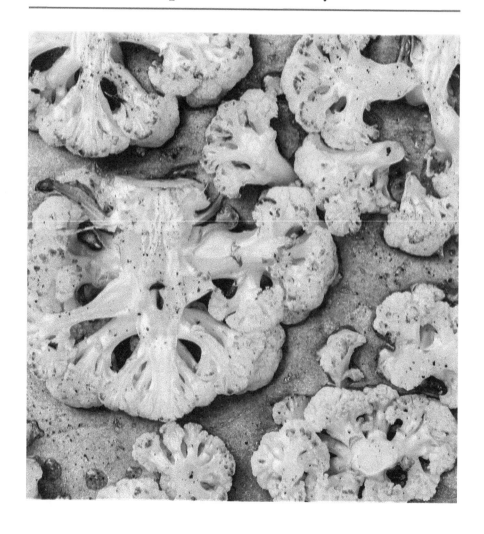

Ingredients

1 head cauliflower
½ lemon, juiced
½ tablespoon olive oil
1 teaspoon curry powder
Sea salt and black pepper to taste

Directions

1. Prepare your cauliflower by washing and removing the leaves and core. Slice it into florets of comparable size.

2. Grease your air fryer with oil and preheat it for 2 minutes at 390° F.

3. Combine fresh lemon juice and curry powder, add the cauliflower florets and stir. Use salt and pepper as seasoning and stir again.

4. Cook for 20 minutes and serve warm.

18. EGGPLANT PARMESAN PANINI

Cal.: 267 | Fat: 11.3g | Protein: 8.5g

Preparation Time: 25 minutes
Cooking Time: 15 minutes
Servings: 2
Requirements: Air fryer

Ingredients

1 medium eggplant, cut into ½ inch slices
½ cup mayonnaise
2 tablespoons milk
Black pepper to taste
½ teaspoon garlic powder
½ teaspoon onion powder
1 tablespoon dried parsley
½ teaspoon Italian seasoning
½ cup breadcrumbs
Sea salt to taste
Fresh basil, chopped for garnishing
¾ cup tomato sauce
2 tablespoons parmesan, grated cheese
2 cups grated mozzarella cheese
2 tablespoons olive oil
4 slices artisan Italian bread
Cooking spray

1. Cover both sides of eggplant with salt. Place them between sheets of paper towels. Set aside for 30 minutes to get rid of excess moisture.

2. In a mixing bowl, combine Italian seasoning, breadcrumbs, parsley, onion powder, garlic powder and season with salt and pepper. In another small bowl, whisk mayonnaise and milk until smooth.

3. Preheat your air fryer to 400° F. Remove the excess salt from eggplant slices. Cover both sides of eggplant with mayonnaise mixture. Press the eggplant slices into the breadcrumb mixture. Use cooking spray on both sides of eggplant slices.

4. Air fry slices in batches for 15 minutes, turning over when halfway done. Each bread slice must be greased with olive oil. On a cutting board, place two slices of bread with oiled sides down. Layer mozzarella cheese and grated parmesan cheese. Place eggplant on cheese. Cover with tomato sauce and add remaining mozzarella and parmesan cheeses.

5. Garnish with chopped fresh basil. Put the second slice of bread oiled side up on top. Take preheated Panini press and place sandwiches on it. Close the lid and cook for 10 minutes.

6. Slice panini into halves and serve.

19. AVOCADO FRIES

Cal.: 263 | Fat: 7.4g | Protein: 8.2g

Preparation Time: 10 minutes
Cooking Time: 15 minutes
Servings: 4
Requirements: Air fryer

Ingredients

1 ounce Aquafina
1 avocado, sliced
½ teaspoon salt
½ cup panko breadcrumbs

Directions

1. Toss the panko breadcrumbs and salt together in a bowl.

2. Pour Aquafina into another bowl. Dredge the avocado slices in Aquafina and then panko breadcrumbs. Arrange the slices in a single layer in an air fryer basket.

3. Air fry at 390° F for 10 minutes.

20. HONEY ROASTED CARROTS

Cal.: 257 | Fat: 11.6g | Protein: 7.3g

Preparation Time: 12 minutes
Cooking Time: 15 minutes
Servings: 2
Requirements: Air fryer

Ingredients

1 tablespoon honey
Salt and pepper to taste
3 cups of baby carrots
1 tablespoon olive oil

Directions

1. In a mixing bowl, combine carrots, honey, and olive oil.

2. Season with salt and pepper.

3. Cook in an air fryer at 390° F for 12 minutes.

21. GARLIC BUTTER SALMON

Cal.: 172 | Fat: 12.3g | Protein: 15.6g

Preparation Time: 10 minutes
Cooking Time: 30 minutes
Servings: 8

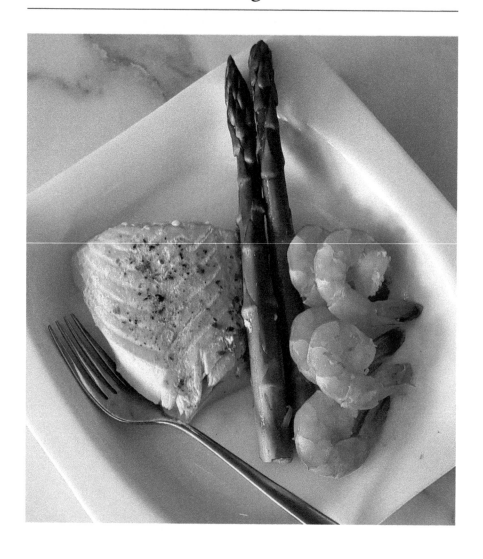

Ingredients

Kosher salt and black pepper, to taste
1 pound (3 pounds) salmon fillet, skin removed
4 tablespoons butter, melted
2 garlic cloves, minced
¼ cup parmesan cheese, freshly grated

Directions

1. Preheat the oven to 3500F and lightly grease a large baking sheet.

2. Season the salmon with salt and black pepper and transfer to the baking sheet.

3. Mix together butter, garlic and parmesan cheese in a small bowl.

4. Marinate salmon in this mixture for about 1 hour.

5. Transfer to the oven and bake for about 25 minutes.

6. Additionally, broil for about 2 minutes until the top becomes lightly golden.

7. Dish out onto a platter and serve hot.

22. TUSCAN BUTTER SALMON

Cal.: 382 | Fat: 27.5g | Protein: 34g

Preparation Time: 15 minutes
Cooking Time: 20 minutes
Servings: 4

Ingredients

4 (6 oz) salmon fillets, patted dry with paper towels
3 tablespoons butter
¾ cup heavy cream
Kosher salt and black pepper
2 cups baby spinach

Directions

1. Season the salmon with salt and black pepper.

2. Heat 1½ tablespoons butter over medium high heat in a large skillet and add salmon skin side up.

3. Cook for about 10 minutes on both sides until deeply golden and dish out onto a plate. Heat the rest of the butter in the skillet and add spinach.

4. Cook for about 5 minutes and stir in the heavy cream.

5. Reduce heat to low and simmer for about 3 minutes.

6. Return the salmon to the skillet and mix well with the sauce.

7. Allow to simmer for about 3 minutes until salmon is cooked through.

8. Dish out and serve hot.

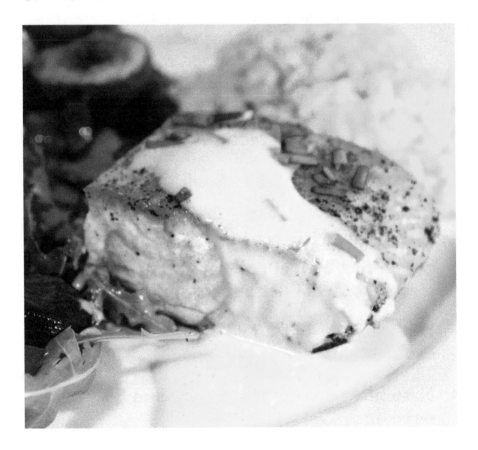

23. MAHI STEW

Cal.: 398 | Fat: 12.5g | Protein: 62.3g

Preparation Time: 15 minutes
Cooking Time: 30 minutes
Servings: 3
Requirements: Pressure cooker

Ingredients

2 tablespoons butter
2 pounds Mahi fillets, cubed
1 onion, chopped
Salt and black pepper, to taste
2 cups homemade fish broth

Directions

1. Season the Mahi fillets with salt and black pepper.

2. Heat butter in a pressure cooker and add onion. Sauté for about 3 minutes and stir in the seasoned Mahi fillets and fish broth.

3. Lock the lid and cook on High Pressure for about 30 minutes.

4. Naturally release the pressure and dish out to serve hot.

24. SOUR CREAM TILAPIA

Cal.: 300 | Fat: 17.9g | Protein: 31.8g

Preparation Time: 10 minutes
Cooking Time: 3 hours
Servings: 3
Requirements: Slow cooker

Ingredients

¾ cup homemade chicken broth
1 pound tilapia fillets
1 cup sour cream
Salt and black pepper, to taste
1 teaspoon cayenne pepper

Directions

1. Put tilapia fillets in the slow cooker along with the rest of the ingredients.

2. Cover the lid and cook on low for about 3 hours.

3. Dish out and serve hot.

25. TILAPIA WITH HERBED BUTTER

Cal.: 281 | Fat: 10.4g | Protein: 38.7g

Preparation Time: 35 minutes
Cooking Time: 25 minutes
Servings: 6
Requirements: Pressure cooker/Instant pot

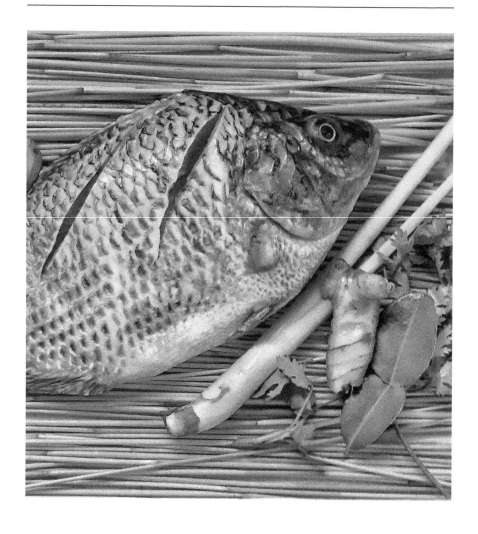

Ingredients

2 pounds tilapia fillets
12 garlic cloves, chopped finely
6 green broccoli, chopped
2 cups herbed butter
Salt and black pepper, to taste

Directions

1. Season the tilapia fillets with salt and black pepper.

2. Put the seasoned tilapia along with all other ingredients in an Instant Pot and mix well.

3. Cover the lid and cook on High Pressure for about 25 minutes.

4. Dish out on a platter and serve hot.

26. ROASTED TROUT

Cal.: 349 | Fat: 28.2g | Protein: 23.3g

Preparation Time: 10 minutes
Cooking Time: 35 minutes
Servings: 4

Ingredients

½ cup fresh lemon juice
1 pound trout fish fillets
4 tablespoons butter
Salt and black pepper, to taste
1 teaspoon dried rosemary, crushed

Directions

1. Put ½ pound trout fillets in a dish and sprinkle with lemon juice and dried rosemary.

2. Season with salt and black pepper and transfer into a skillet.

3. Add butter and cook, covered on medium low heat for about 35 minutes.

4. Dish out the fillets in a platter and serve with a sauce.

27. SOUR FISH WITH HERBED BUTTER

Cal.: 234 | Fat: 11.8g | Protein: 31.5g

Preparation Time: 45 minutes
Cooking Time: 30 minutes
Servings: 3

Ingredients

2 tablespoons herbed butter
3 cod fillets
1 tablespoon vinegar
Salt and black pepper, to taste
½ tablespoon lemon pepper seasoning

Directions

1. Preheat the oven to 3750F and grease a baking tray. Mix together cod fillets, vinegar, lemon pepper seasoning, salt and black pepper in a bowl.

2. Marinate for about 3 hours and then arrange on the baking tray.

3. Transfer into the oven and bake for about 30 minutes. Remove from the oven and serve with herbed butter.

28. COD COCONUT CURRY

Cal.: 223 | Fat: 6.1g | Protein: 35.5g

Preparation Time: 35 minutes
Cooking Time: 25 minutes
Servings: 6

Ingredients

1 onion, chopped
2 pounds cod
1 cup dry coconut, chopped
Salt and black pepper, to taste
1 cup fresh lemon juice

Directions

1. Put the cod along with all other ingredients in a pressure cooker.

2. Add 2 cups of water and cover the lid.

3. Cook on High Pressure for about 25 minutes and naturally release the pressure.

4. Open the lid and dish out the curry to serve hot.

29. GARLIC SHRIMP WITH GOAT CHEESE

Cal.: 294 | Fat: 15g | Protein: 35.8g

Preparation Time: 30 minutes
Cooking Time: 20 minutes
Servings: 4

Ingredients

4 tablespoons herbed butter
Salt and black pepper, to taste
1 pound large raw shrimp
4 ounces goat cheese
4 garlic cloves, chopped

Directions

1. Preheat the oven to 3750F and grease a baking dish.

2. Mix together herbed butter, garlic, raw shrimp, salt and black pepper in a bowl.

3. Put the marinated shrimp on the baking dish and top with the shredded cheese.

4. Place in the oven and bake for about 25 minutes. Take the shrimp out and serve hot.

30. ZUPPA TOSCANA WITH CAULIFLOWER

Cal.: 653 | Fat: 26g | Protein: 4g

Preparation Time: 5 minutes
Cooking Time: 25 minutes
Servings: 4
Requirements: Pressure cooker

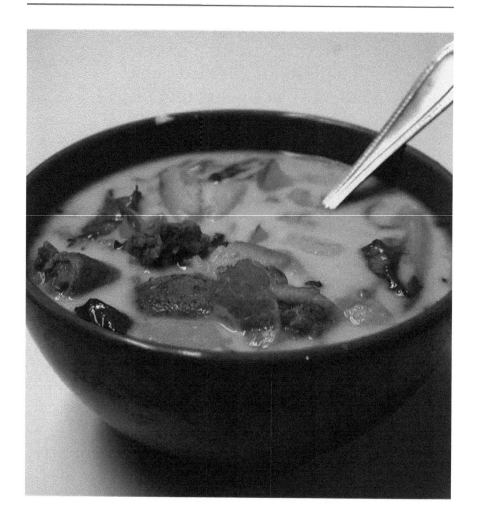

Ingredients

1 lb. ground Italian sausage
6 cups homemade low-sodium chicken stock
2 cups cauliflower florets - 1 onion, finely
chopped
1 cup kale, stemmed and roughly chopped
1 (14.5-ounce) can of full-fat coconut milk
¼ tsp. sea salt
¼ tsp. freshly cracked black pepper

Directions

1. On the Instant Pot, press "Sauté" and add the Italian ground sausage. Cook until brown, stirring occasionally and breaking up the meat with a wooden spoon.

2. Add the remaining ingredients except for the kale and coconut milk and stir until well combined.

3. Cover and cook for 10 minutes on high pressure. When done, release the pressure naturally and remove the lid. Stir in the kale and coconut milk.

4. Cover and sit for 5 minutes or until the kale has wilted.

5. Serve and enjoy!

31. GRAIN FREE SALMON BREAD

Cal.: 413 | Fat: 32.4g | Protein: 31.8g

Preparation Time: 15 minutes
Cooking Time: 20 minutes
Servings: 6

Ingredients

½ cup olive oil
¼ teaspoon baking soda
½ cup coconut milk
2 pounds salmon, steamed and shredded
2 pastured eggs

Directions

1. Preheat the oven to 3750F and grease a baking dish with olive oil.

2. Mix together coconut milk, eggs, baking soda and salmon in a bowl.

3. Pour the batter of salmon bread in the baking dish and transfer into the oven.

4. Bake for about 20 minutes and remove from the oven to serve hot.

32. CHEESY TUNA PESTO PASTA

Cal.: 696 | Fat: 27g | Protein: 40g

Preparation Time: 10 minutes
Cooking Time: 25 minutes
Servings: 4

Ingredients

4 cups zucchini noodles, spiralized, cooked
1 cup cheddar, grated
1 cup yellowfin tuna in olive oil
7 oz. basil pesto
1½ cup punnet cherry tomato, halved

Directions

1. Mix pesto and tuna with oil in a bowl. Mash well. Add in 1/3 of the cheese and add all the tomatoes.

2. Add noodles to the bowl, toss well to coat. Transfer the mixture to a baking dish and add the remaining cheese on top.

3. Broil the dish for 4 minutes. Serve.

33. GARLIC BUTTER BEEF STEAK

Cal.: 337 | Fat: 18.7g | Protein: 34.5g

Preparation Time: 5 minutes
Cooking Time: 15 minutes
Servings: 2
Requirements: Pressure cooker

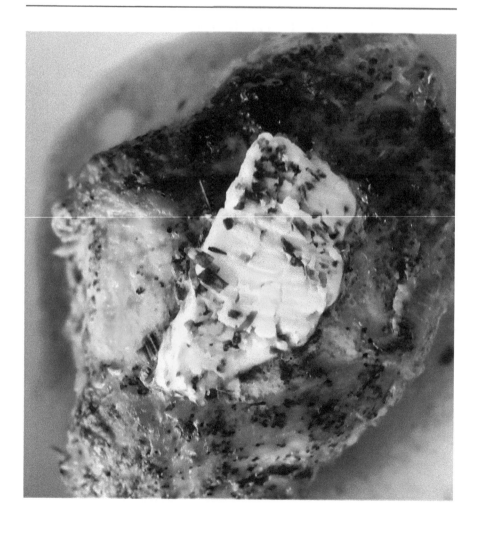

Ingredients

1 lb. beef sirloin steaks
½ cup red wine
4 tbsps. unsalted butter
2 tbsps. fresh parsley, finely chopped
4 medium garlic cloves, peeled and minced
Fine sea salt and freshly cracked black pepper

Directions

1. Season the beef steaks with sea salt and freshly cracked black pepper.

2. On the Instant Pot, press "Sauté" and add the butter. Once melted, add the beef steaks and sear for 2 minutes per side or until brown.

3. Pour in the red wine and fresh parsley. Cover and cook for 12 minutes on high pressure. When done, release the pressure naturally and carefully remove the lid.

4. Top the steak with the butter sauce. Serve and enjoy!

34. INSTANT POT TERIYAKI CHICKEN

Cal.: 259 | Fat: 24.3g | Protein: 2.3g

Preparation Time: 5 minutes
Cooking Time: 35 minutes
Servings: 4
Requirements: Pressure cooker

Ingredients

1/2 cup soy sauce
1/2 cup water
1/2 cup brown sugar
2 tbsps. rice wine vinegar
1 tbsp. mirin (Japanese sweet wine)
1 tbsp. sake
1 tbsp. minced garlic
1 dash freshly cracked black pepper
1 lb. skinless, boneless chicken

Directions

1. Combine soy sauce, brown sugar, water, rice wine vinegar, sake, mirin, pepper, and garlic in a bowl to prepare the sauce.

2. Put chicken in an electric pressure cooker (such as Instant Pot(R)). Pour the sauce over.

3. Close lid and lock. Set to Meat function, with the timer on to 12 minutes. Give 10-15 minutes for pressure to build.

4. Gently release pressure with the quick-release method according to manufacturer's Directions, for 5 minutes. Remove the lid. Insert the instant-read thermometer into the middle of the chicken and make sure to reach at least 165°F (74°C). If not hot enough, cook for 2-4 more minutes.

5. Take chicken out from the cooker. Shred or cut up. Mix with sauce from the pot.

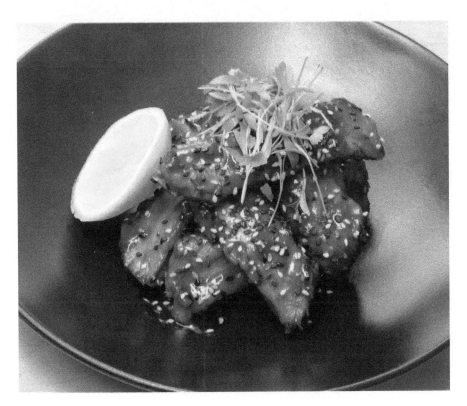

35. TERIYAKI SALMON

Cal.: 93 | Fat: 4g | Protein: 13g

Preparation Time: 15 minutes
Cooking Time: 5 minutes
Servings: 2

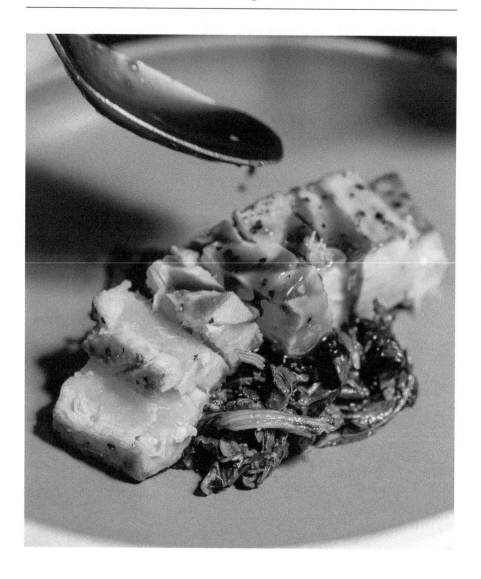

Ingredients

3 tbsps. lime juice
2 tbsps. olive oil
2 tbsps. reduced-sodium teriyaki sauce
1 tbsp. balsamic vinegar
1 tbsp. Dijon mustard
1 tsp. garlic powder
6 drops hot pepper sauce
6 uncooked jumbo salmon

Directions

1. Mix together all ingredients except the salmon in a big zip-lock plastic bag, then put in the shrimp. Seal the zip lock bag and turn to coat the salmon. Keep in the fridge for an hour and occasionally turn.

2. Drain the marinated salmon and discard marinade. Broil the salmon 4 inches from heat for 3 to 4 minutes per side or until the salmon turn pink in color.

36. SPICY OVEN BAKED CHICKEN

Cal.: 248 | Fat: 27g | Protein: 2g

Preparation Time: 10 minutes
Cooking Time: 23 minutes
Servings: 4

Ingredients

4 tablespoons of fat-free buttermilk
2 tablespoons of spicy brown mustard
2 lean chicken breasts
¼ cup of whole wheat breadcrumbs
¼ cup chopped walnuts
1 tablespoon of chopped rosemary
¼ tsp of salt
½ tsp of pepper
½ tsp of cayenne pepper
2 tablespoons of honey

Directions

1. Set your oven for 425 degrees.

2. While your oven warms up, get out a medium sized mixing bowl and add your 4 tablespoons of fat-free buttermilk and your 2 tablespoons of spicy brown mustard.

3. Now place each chicken breast into the bowl, and turn them over in the mixture, until they are thoroughly coated.

4. Next, place a frying pan onto a burner set for high heat and add your ¼ cup of wheat breadcrumbs to the pan, followed by your ¼ cup of chopped walnuts, your 1 tablespoon of chopped rosemary, your ¼ tsp of salt, your ½ tsp of pepper, and your ½ tsp of cayenne pepper and stir everything together well as they cook over the next 2 to 3 minutes before turning the burner off.

5. Now place your buttermilk coated chicken into the pan and flip it around in the cooked breadcrumb ingredients until they are thoroughly coated with it as well.

6. Place your breadcrumb coated chicken breasts in an oven safe dish and cook for about 20 minutes.

7. Serve when ready.

37. LEAN GREEN SOUP

Cal.: 182 | Fat: 10g | Protein: 8g

Preparation Time: 3 minutes
Cooking Time: 9 minutes
Servings: 4

Ingredients

500 ml vegetable stock
1 tablespoon of coconut oil
1 tablespoon of minced garlic
2 tablespoons of water
1 tsp of coriander
1 tsp of turmeric
½ cup of chopped broccoli
½ cup of chopped kale
½ cup of chopped parsley

Directions

1. Add your tablespoon of coconut oil to a saucepan followed by your tablespoon of minced garlic, your tsp of coriander, and your tsp of turmeric.

2. Set the burner on high and add 2 tablespoons of water to the mix.

3. Stir ingredients together as they cook over the next 2 minutes.

4. Now add your 500 ml vegetable stock followed by your ½ cup of chopped broccoli, your ½ cup of chopped kale, and your ½ cup of chopped parsley.

5. Stir everything together well and allow to cook for another 7 minutes.

6. Allow to cool slightly, and serve when ready.

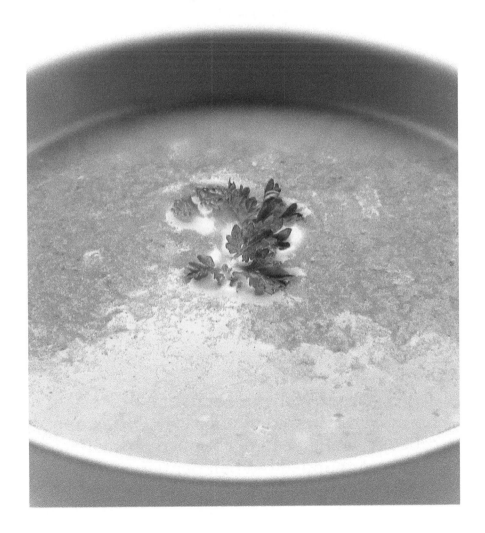

38. BROWN RICE STIR FRY

Cal.: 197 | Fat: 8g | Protein: 6g

Preparation Time: 2 minutes
Cooking Time: 5 minutes
Servings: 4

Ingredients

1 cup of brown (cooked) rice
2 cups of chopped cabbage
½ cup of chopped broccoli
¼ cup of chopped red bell pepper
¼ cup of chopped zucchini
2 tablespoons of olive oil
1 tablespoon of chopped garlic
1 tablespoon of chopped parsley
¼ tsp of cayenne powder
1 tablespoon of soy sauce
1 tsp of sesame seeds
2 cups of water

Directions

1. To get started, add your 2 cups of water to a large frying pan followed by your 2 cups of chopped cabbage, your ½ cup of chopped broccoli, your ¼ cup of chopped red bell pepper, and your ¼ cup of chopped zucchini.

2. Set the burner on high and stir and cook over the next 3 minutes.

3. After this, drain any left-over water from the pan before setting it to the side.

4. Now place a wok (or similar cooking pan) onto a burner set for high heat and add your 2 tablespoons of olive oil, your tablespoon of chopped garlic, your tablespoon of chopped parsley, and cook for about 1 minute.

5. Next, add in your cooked vegetables followed by your cup of cooked rice, and stir and cook everything together for about a minute.

6. Drizzle your tablespoon of soy sauce, followed by your tsp of sesame seeds on top.

7. Serve when ready.

39. LOW CARB CABBAGE BOWL

Cal.: 327 | Fat: 18g | Protein: 7g

Preparation Time: 3 minutes
Cooking Time: 14 minutes
Servings: 4

Ingredients

2 tablespoons of olive oil
½ cup of chopped carrots
¼ cup of diced onions
½ tsp of salt
½ tsp of pepper
1 tsp of cumin
½ tsp of turmeric
1 cup of shredded cabbage
1 cup of chopped potatoes

Directions

1. Place a medium sized saucepan onto a burner set for high heat and add your 2 tablespoons of olive oil to the pan.

2. Next, add your ½ cup of chopped carrots, your ¼ cup of diced onions, your ½ tsp of salt, and your ½ tsp of pepper.

3. Stir and cook these ingredients for about 4 minutes before adding your cup of shredded cabbage, and your cup of chopped potatoes, followed by your tsp of cumin and your ½ tsp of turmeric.

4. Continue to stir and cook your ingredients for about 10 more minutes.

5. Turn the burner off, allow food to cool for a moment and serve.

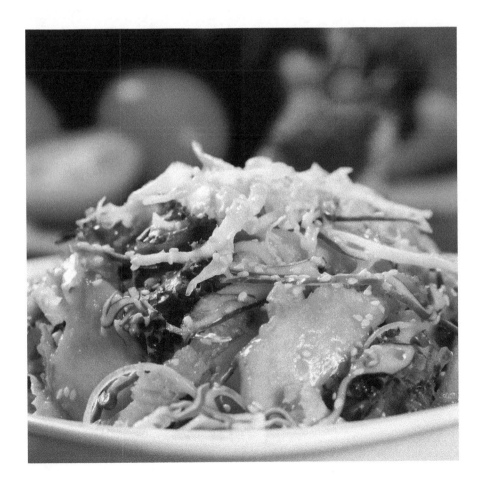

40. GARLIC HERB GRILLED CHICKEN BREAST

Cal.: 187 | Fat: 6g | Protein: 32g

Preparation Time: 7 minutes
Cooking Time: 20 minutes
Servings: 4

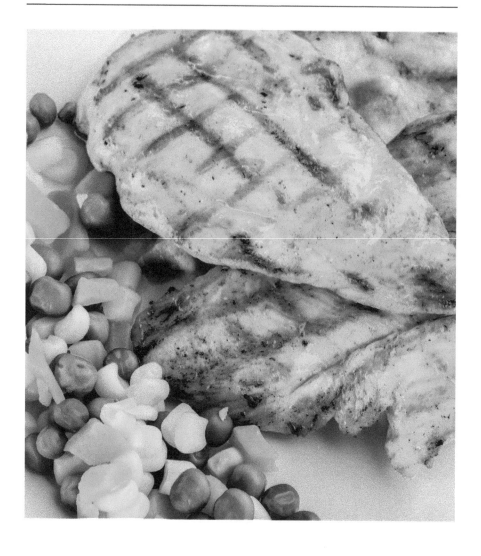

Ingredients

1¼ pounds Chicken Breasts, skinless and
boneless
2 teaspoons Olive oil
1 tablespoon Garlic & Herb Seasoning Blend
Salt
Pepper

Directions

1. Pat dry the chicken breasts, coat it with olive oil and season it with salt and pepper on both sides.

2. Season the chicken with garlic and herb seasoning or any other seasoning of your choice.

3. Turn the grill on and oil the grate.

4. Place the chicken on the hot grate and let it grill till the sides turn white.

5. Flip them over and let it cook again.

6. When the internal temperature is about 160 degree, it is most likely cooked.

7. Set aside for 15 minutes. Chop into pieces

41. CAJUN SHRIMP

Cal.: 127 | Fat: 10g | Protein: 7g

Preparation Time: 10 minutes
Cooking Time: 5 minutes
Servings: 2

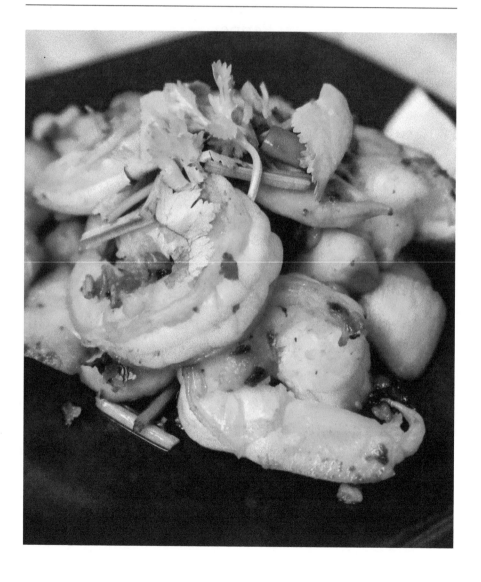

Ingredients

16 Tiger shrimp
2 tablespoons Cornstarch
1 teaspoon Cayenne pepper
1 teaspoon Old bay seasoning
Salt
Pepper
1 teaspoon Olive oil

Directions

1. Rinse the shrimp. Pat dry.

2. In a bowl, combine corn starch, cayenne pepper, old bay seasoning, salt, pepper. Stir.

3. In a bowl, add the shrimp. Drizzle olive oil over shrimp to lightly coat.

4. Dip the shrimp in seasoning, shake off any excess.

5. Preheat fryer to 375°F. Lightly spray the cook basket with non-stick Keto cooking spray.

6. Transfer to fryer. Cook for 5 minutes; shake after 2 minutes, until cooked thoroughly.

7. Serve on a platter.

42. SESAME-CRUSTED MAHI-MAHI

Cal.: 282 | Fat: 17g | Protein: 18g

Preparation Time: 5 minutes
Cooking Time: 13 minutes
Servings: 4

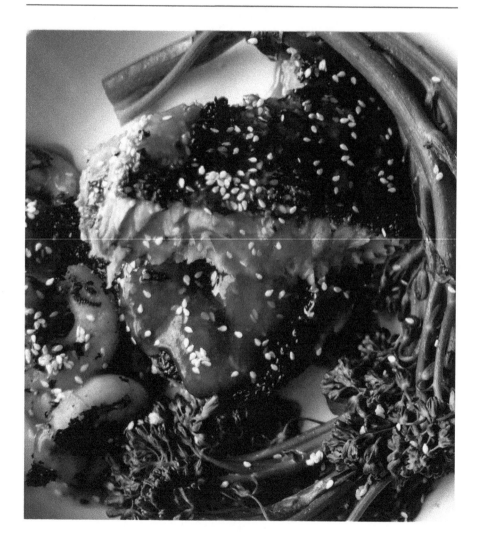

Ingredients

2 tablespoons Dijon mustard
1 tablespoon Sour cream, low-fat
½ cup Sesame seeds
2 tablespoons Olive oil
1 Lemon, wedged
4 (4 oz. each) Mahi-mahi or sole filets

Directions

1. Rinse filets and pat dry. In a bowl, mix sour cream and mustard. Spread this mixture on all sides of fish. Roll in sesame seeds to coat.

2. Heat olive oil in a large skillet over medium heat. Pan-fry fish, turning once, for 5–8 minutes or until fish flakes when tested with fork and sesame seeds are toasted. Serve immediately with lemon wedges.

43. COUNTRY CHICKEN

Cal.: 480 | Fat: 26g | Protein: 36g

Preparation Time: 10 minutes
Cooking Time: 15 minutes
Servings: 2

Ingredients

¾ pound Chicken tenders, fresh, boneless
skinless
½ cup Almond meal
½ cup Almond flour
1 teaspoon Rosemary, dried
Salt
Pepper
2 Eggs, beaten

Directions

1. Rinse the chicken tenders, pat dry.

2. In a medium bowl, pour in almond flour.

3. In a medium bowl, beat the eggs.

4. In a separate bowl, pour in almond meal. Season with rosemary, salt, pepper.

5. Take the chicken pieces and toast in flour, then

egg, then almond meal. Set on a tray.

6. Place the tray in the freezer for 5 minutes.

7. Preheat fryer to 350°F. Lightly spray the cook basket with non-stick cooking spray.

8. Cook tenders for 10 minutes. After the timer runs out, set the temperature to 390°F, cook 5 more minutes until golden brown.

9. Serve on a platter. Side with preferred dipping sauce.

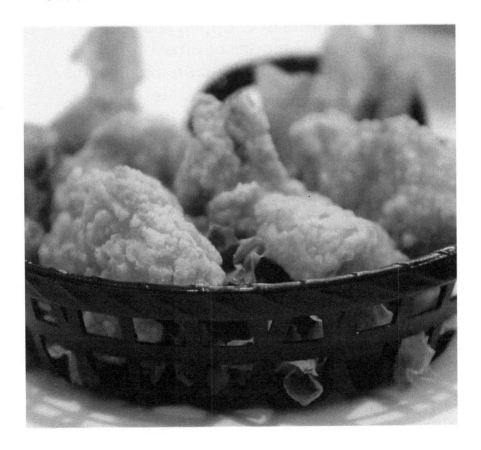

44. PORTOBELLO MUSHROOM FAJITA WRAPS

Cal.: 207 | Fat: 2g | Protein: 7g

Preparation Time: 10 minutes
Cooking Time: 15 minutes
Servings: 3

Ingredients

3 corn tortillas
1 tablespoon of chopped jalapenos
2 tablespoons of olive oil
1 cup of chopped portobello mushrooms
¼ cup of chopped onions
¼ cup of chopped bell peppers
1 tablespoon of chopped garlic
1 tsp of cumin
1 tsp of smoked paprika
¼ tsp of salt

Directions

1. Get out a large pan and place it onto a burner set for high heat before adding your tablespoon of chopped jalapenos, your ¼ cup of chopped onions, your ¼ cup of chopped bell peppers, your tsp of cumin, your tsp of smoked paprika, and your tablespoon of chopped garlic.

2. Stir and cook all of your ingredients together for about 2 minutes.

3. After this, add your cup of chopped mushrooms.

4. Continue to stir and cook your ingredients over the next 10 minutes.

5. Evenly distribute your cooked ingredients into your tortillas and wrap them up.

6. This dish is ready to eat!

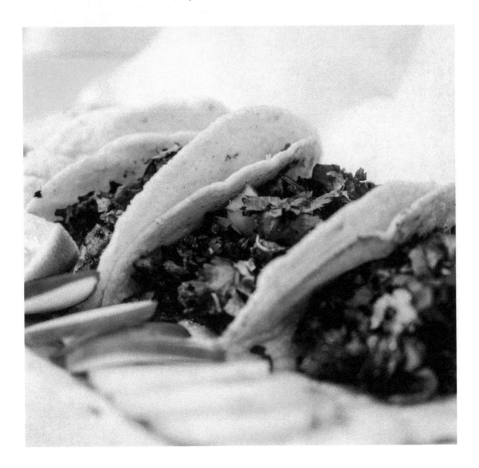

45. MAHI-MAHI TACOS WITH AVOCADO AND FRESH CABBAGE

Cal.: 251 | Fat: 9g | Protein: 25g

Preparation Time: 5 minutes
Cooking Time: 15 minutes
Servings: 4

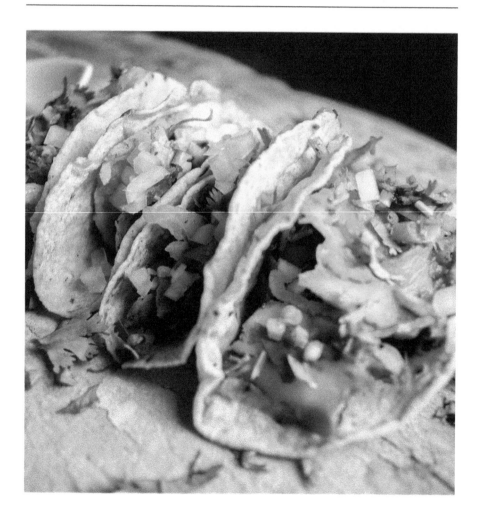

Ingredients

1 pound Mahi-mahi
Salt
Pepper
1 teaspoon Olive oil
1 Avocado
4 Corn tortillas
2 cups Cabbage, shredded
2 Quartered limes

Directions

1. Season fish with salt and pepper.

2. Set a pan over medium-high heat. Add in oil and heat. Once the oil is hot, sauté fish for about 3–4 minutes on each side. Slice or flake fish into 1-ounce pieces.

3. Slice avocado in half. Remove seed and, using a spoon, remove the flesh from the skin. Slice the avocado halves into ½ thick slices.

4. In a small pan, warm corn tortillas; cook for about 1 minute on each side. Place one-fourth of Mahi-mahi on each tortilla, top with avocado and cabbage. Serve with lime wedges.

46. BALSAMIC CHICKEN WITH ROASTED VEGETABLES

Cal.: 450 | Fat: 17g | Protein: 48g

Preparation Time: 10 minutes
Cooking Time: 30 minutes
Servings: 4

Ingredients

10 asparaguses, ends trimmed and cut in half
8 boneless, skinless chicken thighs, fat trimmed
2 bell peppers, sliced into strips
½ cup carrots, sliced into half long and cut into
3-inch pieces
1 red onion, chopped into large chunks
¼ cup + 1 tablespoon balsamic vinegar
5 oz. mushrooms, sliced
2 tablespoons olive oil
½ tablespoon dried oregano
2 sage leaves, chopped
2 garlic cloves, smashed and chopped
½ teaspoon sugar
1½ tablespoons rosemary
1 teaspoon salt
Black pepper, to taste
Cooking spray

Directions

1. Preheat the oven to 425°F.

2. Season chicken with salt and pepper and spray 2 large baking sheets with cooking spray.

3. Mix all the ingredients in a bowl and mix well. Place everything on the prepared baking sheet and spread it in a single layer.

4. Bake for 25 minutes. Serve.

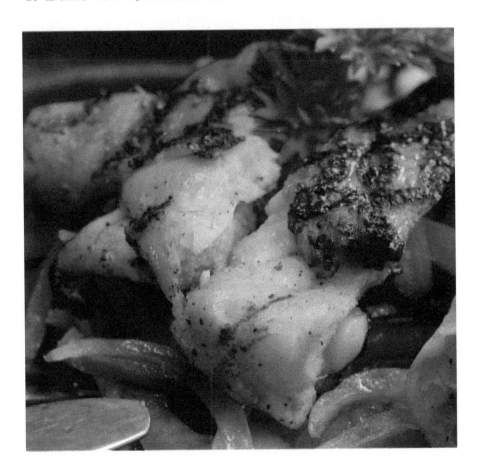

47. LOW CARB CHILI

Cal.: 348 | Fat: 28.8g | Protein: 14.9g

Preparation Time: 5 minutes
Cooking Time: 40 minutes
Servings: 6

Ingredients

1 bell pepper, chopped
1¼ lb. ground beef
8 oz. tomato paste
1½ tomato, chopped
2 celery sticks, chopped
½ cup onion, chopped
1½ teaspoons cumin
¾ cup of water
1½ teaspoon chili powder
1½ teaspoons salt
½ teaspoon pepper

Directions

1. Cook the meat in a frying pan until brown. Drain the excess fat and season meat with salt.

2. Add peppers and onions to the pan and cook for 2 minutes. Mix onions, cooked meat, peppers,

tomatoes, water, celery, and tomato paste in a pot.

3. Add the spices to the pot. Bring to a boil and reduce the heat to low-medium. Cook for 2 hours while stirring every 30 minutes. Serve.

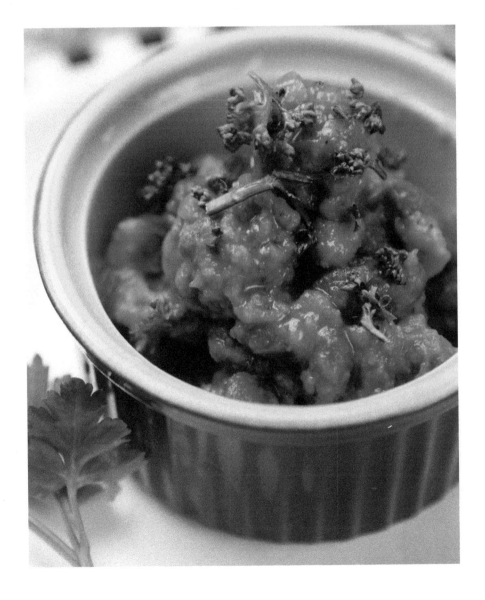

48. KETO MEATLOAF

Cal.: 344 | Fat: 29g | Protein: 33g

Preparation Time: 15 minutes
Cooking Time: 1 hour
Servings: 6

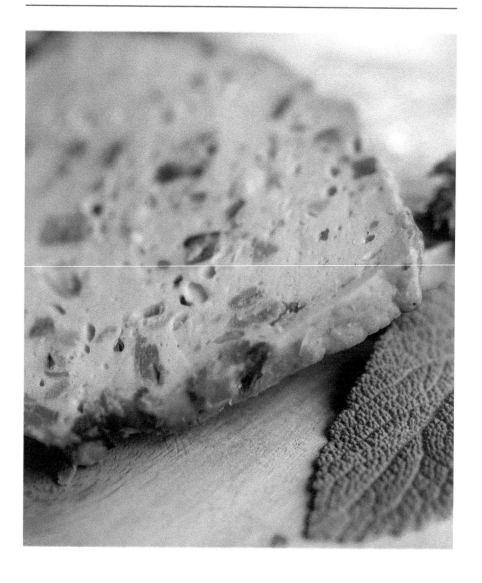

Ingredients

2 eggs
2 lbs. 85% lean grass-fed ground beef
¼ cup nutritional yeast
1 tablespoon lemon zest
2 tablespoons avocado oil
¼ cup parsley, chopped
4 garlic cloves
¼ cup oregano, chopped
½ tablespoon pink Himalayan salt
1 teaspoon black pepper

Directions

1. Preheat the oven to 400°F. Mix beef, yeast, salt, and pepper in a bowl.

2. Mix eggs, oil, garlic, and herbs in a blender and blend until everything is mixed well. Add this mixture to the beef and mix well.

3. Add the beef mixture to a small loaf pan. Arrange the pan on the middle rack and bake for 1 hour. Remove the pan from the oven. Let cool for 10 minutes. Serve.

49. CHICKEN PARMESAN

Cal.: 318 | Fat: 17g | Protein: 36g

Preparation Time: 5 minutes
Cooking Time: 19 minutes
Servings: 8

Ingredients

2 lbs. boneless skinless chicken breast
4 oz. fresh mozzarella
1/3 cup sugar-free marinara
1 cup almond flour
1 cup parmesan cheese, grated
2 eggs
1 teaspoon Italian seasoning
½ teaspoon black pepper
½ teaspoon sea salt

Directions

1. Add chicken to a plastic bag and pound until about ½-inch thick.

2. Add 1 teaspoon Italian seasoning, a cup of parmesan cheese, ½ teaspoon sea salt, a cup of almond flour, and ½ teaspoon pepper. Mix well.

3. Add eggs to a separate bowl and whisk well. Pat dry the chicken with paper towels.

4. Dip chicken into the egg mixture and then coat with almond flour mixture. Brush with oil or coat with cooking spray.

5. Preheat the oven to 425°F. Place chicken on a baking sheet lined with parchment paper. Cook for about 11-12 minutes.

6. Then flip the chicken, spray with cooking spray and cook for 5 minutes more.

7. Sprinkle each piece with mozzarella and drizzle with pasta sauce. Transfer back to the oven and cook for a few minutes until the cheese is melted.

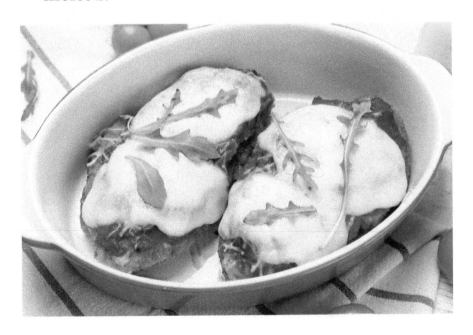

50. MUSHROOM BACON SKILLET

Cal.: 313 | Fat: 13.6g | Protein: 8.5g

Preparation Time: 5 minutes
Cooking Time: 10 minutes
Servings: 1

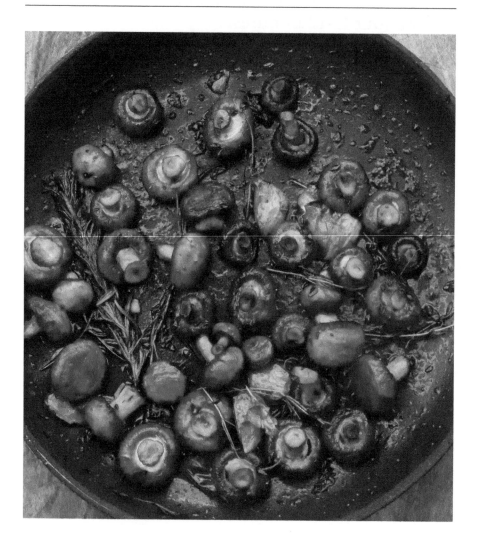

Ingredients

½ teaspoon salt
1 tablespoon garlic, minced
4 slices pastured pork bacon, cut into ½-inch
pieces
2 sprigs thyme, leaves only
2 cups mushrooms, halved

Directions

1. Preheat a skillet over medium heat. Add bacon and cook until crispy. Remove from the pan.

2. Add sliced mushrooms. Sauté until softened, stirring often.

3. Add garlic, thyme, and salt. Cook for 5 minutes more, stirring often.

4. When mushrooms become golden, turn the heat off.

5. Garnish mushroom bacon with greens and enjoy!

Cooking Conversion

TEMPERATURE CONVERSIONS	
CELSIUS	**FAHRENHEIT**
54.5°C	130°F
60.0°C	140°F
65.5°C	150°F
71.1°C	160°F
76.6°C	170°F
82.2°C	180°F
87.8°C	190°F
93.3°C	200°F
100°C	212°F

WEIGHT COVERSION	
½ oz.	15g
1 oz.	30g
2 oz.	60g
3 oz.	85g
4 oz.	110g
5 oz.	140g
6 oz.	170g
7 oz.	200g
8 oz.	225g
9 oz.	255g
10 oz.	280g
11 oz.	310g
12 oz.	340g
13 oz.	370g
14 oz.	400g
15 oz.	425g
1 lb.	450g

LIQUID VOLUME CONVERSION		
CUPS / TABLE-SPOONS	**FL. OUNCES**	**MILLILITERS**
1 cup	8 fl. Oz.	240 ml
¾ cup	6 fl. Oz.	180 ml
2/3 cup	5 fl. Oz.	150 ml
½ cup	4 fl. Oz.	120 ml
1/3 cup	2 ½ fl. Oz.	75 ml
¼ cup	2 fl. Oz.	60 ml
1/8 cup	1 fl. Oz.	30 ml
1 tablespoon	½ fl. Oz.	15 ml

TEASPOON (tsp.) / TABLE-SPOON (Tbsp.)	**MILLILITERS**
1 tsp.	5ml
2 tsp.	10ml
1 Tbsp.	15ml
2 Tbsp.	30ml
3 Tbsp.	45ml
4 Tbsp.	60ml
5 Tbsp.	75ml
6 Tbsp.	90ml
7 Tbsp.	105ml

LIQUID VOLUME MEASUREMENTS

TABLE-SPOONS	TEASPOONS	FLUID OUNCES	CUPS
16	48	8 fl. Oz.	1
12	36	6 fl. Oz.	¾
8	24	4 fl. Oz.	½
5 ½	16	2 2/3 fl. Oz.	1/3
4	12	2 fl. Oz.	¼
1	3	0.5 fl. Oz.	1/16

Recipe Index